Keto Meal Prep for Beginners

Tasty Recipes for Homemade Cooking to Prepare in No Time for Whole Family

Isabelle Lauren

© **Copyright 2021 - All rights reserved.**

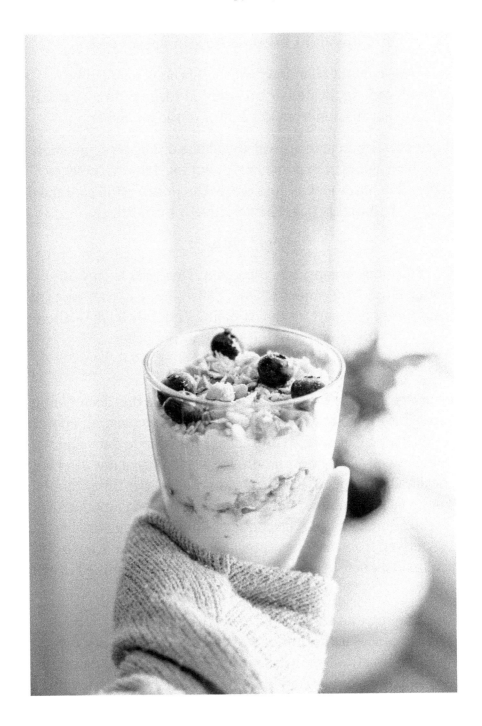

Table of Contents

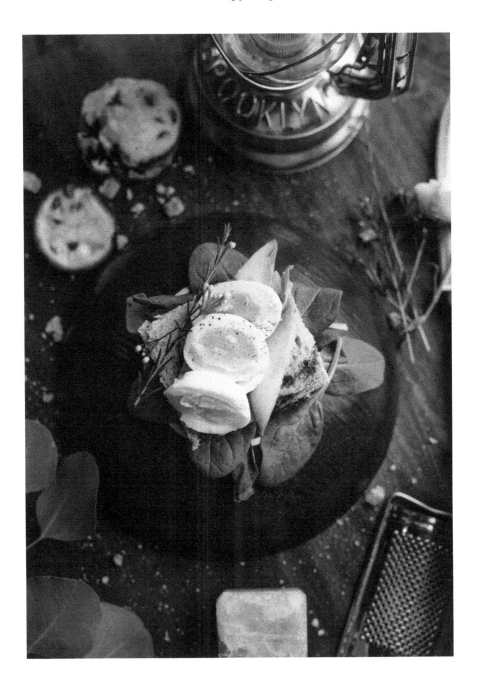

BREAKFAST

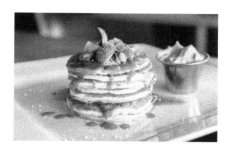

1. Chocolate Cupcakes with Matcha

Preparation Time: 35 minutes

Cooking Time: 0 minutes

Servings: 4

Ingredients:

- 150g / 5 oz. self-rising flour

- 200 g / 7 oz. caster sugar

- 60 g / 2.1 oz. cocoa

- ½ teaspoon. salt

- ½ teaspoon. fine espresso coffee, decaf if preferred

- 120 ml / ½ cup milk

- ½ teaspoon. vanilla extract

- 50 ml / ¼ cup vegetable oil

- 1 egg

- 120 ml / ½ cup of water

- For the icing:

- 50 g / 1.7 oz. butter,

- 50 g / 1.7 oz. icing sugar

- 1 tablespoon matcha green tea powder

- ½ teaspoon vanilla bean paste

- 50 g / 1.7 oz. soft cream cheese

Directions:

1. Heat the oven and Line a cupcake tin with paper

2. Put the flour, sugar, cocoa, salt, and coffee powder in a large bowl and mix well.

3. Add milk, vanilla extract, vegetable oil, and egg to dry ingredients and use an electric mixer to beat until well combined. Gently pour the boiling water slowly and beat on low speed until completely combined. Use the high speed to beat for another minute to add air to the dough. The dough is much more liquid than a normal cake mix. Have faith; It will taste fantastic!

4. Arrange the dough evenly between the cake boxes. Each cake box must not be more than ¾ full. Bake for 15-18 minutes, until the dough resumes when hit. Remove from oven and allow cooling completely before icing.

5. To make the icing, beat your butter and icing sugar until they turn pale and smooth. Add the matcha powder and vanilla and mix again. Add the cream cheese and beat until it is smooth. Pipe or spread on the cakes.

Nutrition: Calories 435 Fat 5 Fiber 3 Carbs 7 Protein 9

2. Sesame Chicken Salad

Preparation Time: 20 minutes

Cooking Time: 0 minutes

Servings: 4

Ingredients:

- 1 tablespoon of sesame seeds

- 1 cucumber, peeled, halved lengthwise, without a teaspoon, and sliced.

- 100 g / 3.5 oz. cabbage, chopped

- 60 g pak choi, finely chopped

- ½ red onion, thinly sliced

- Large parsley (20 g / 0.7 oz.), chopped.

- 150 g / 5 oz. cooked chicken, minced

- For the dressing:

- 1 tablespoon of extra virgin olive oil

- 1 teaspoon of sesame oil

- 1 lime juice

- 1 teaspoon of light honey

- 2 teaspoons soy sauce

Directions:

1. Roast your sesame seeds in a dry pan for 2 minutes until they become slightly golden and fragrant.

2. Transfer to a plate to cool.

3. In a small bowl, mix olive oil, sesame oil, lime juice, honey, and soy sauce to prepare the dressing.

4. Place the cucumber, black cabbage, pak choi, red onion, and parsley in a large bowl and mix gently.

5. Pour over the dressing and mix again.

6. Distribute the salad between two dishes and complete with the shredded chicken. Sprinkle with sesame seeds just before serving.

Nutrition: Calories 345 Fat 5 Fiber 2 Carbs 10 Protein 4

3. Bacon Appetizers

Preparation Time: 15 minutes

Cooking Time: 2 hours

Servings: 6

Ingredients:

- 1 pack Keto crackers

- ¾ cup Parmesan cheese, grated

- 1 lb. bacon, sliced thinly

Directions:

1. Preheat your oven to 250 degrees F.

2. Arrange the crackers on a baking sheet.

3. Sprinkle cheese

4. on top of each cracker.

5. Wrap each cracker with the bacon.

6. Bake in the oven for 2 hours.

Nutrition: Calories 440 Total Fat 33.4g Saturated Fat 11g Cholesterol 86mg Sodium 1813mg Total Carbohydrate 3.7g Dietary Fiber 0.1g Total Sugars 0.1g Protein 29.4g Potassium 432mg

4. Appetizer Skewers

Preparation Time: 10 minutes

Cooking Time: 0 minute

Servings: 6

Ingredients:

- 6 small mozzarella balls

- 1 tablespoon olive oil

- Salt to taste

- 1/8 teaspoon dried oregano

- 2 roasted yellow peppers, sliced into strips and rolled

- 6 cherry tomatoes

- 6 green olives, pitted

- 6 Kalamata olives, pitted

- 2 artichoke hearts, sliced into wedges

- 6 slices salami, rolled

- 6 leaves fresh basil

Directions:

1. Toss the mozzarella balls in olive oil.

2. Season with salt and oregano.

3. Thread the mozzarella balls and the rest of the ingredients into skewers.

4. Serve in a platter.

Nutrition: Calories 180 Total Fat 11.8g Saturated Fat 4.5g Cholesterol 26mg Sodium 482mg Total Carbohydrate 11.7g Dietary Fiber 4.8g Total Sugars 4.1g Protein 9.2g Potassium 538mg

5. Jalapeno Poppers

Preparation Time: 30 minutes

Cooking Time: 60 minutes

Servings: 10

Ingredients:

- 5 fresh jalapenos, sliced and seeded

- 4 oz. package cream cheese

- ¼ lb. bacon, sliced in half

Directions:

1. Preheat your oven to 275 degrees F.

2. Place a wire rack over your baking sheet.

3. Stuff each jalapeno with cream cheese and wrap in bacon.

4. Secure with a toothpick.

5. Place on the baking sheet.

6. Bake for 1 hour and 15 minutes.

Nutrition: Calories 103 Total Fat 8.7g Saturated Fat 4.1g Cholesterol 25mg Sodium 296mg Total Carbohydrate 0.9g Dietary Fiber 0.2g Total Sugars 0.3g Protein 5.2g Potassium 93mg

6. BLT Party Bites

Preparation Time: 35 minutes

Cooking Time: 0 minute **Servings: 8**

Ingredients:

- 4 oz. bacon, chopped

- 3 tablespoons panko breadcrumbs

- 1 tablespoon Parmesan cheese, grated

- 1 teaspoon mayonnaise

- 1 teaspoon lemon juice

- Salt to taste ½ heart Romaine lettuce, shredded

- 6 cocktail tomatoes

Directions:

1. Put the bacon in a pan over medium heat.

2. Fry until crispy.

3. Transfer bacon to a plate lined with paper towel.

4. Add breadcrumbs and cook until crunchy.

5. Transfer breadcrumbs to another plate also lined with paper towel.

6. Sprinkle Parmesan cheese on top of the breadcrumbs.

7. Mix the mayonnaise, salt and lemon juice.

8. Toss the Romaine in the mayo mixture.

9. Slice each tomato on the bottom to create a flat surface so it can stand by itself. Slice the top off as well.

10. Scoop out the insides of the tomatoes.

11. Stuff each tomato with the bacon, Parmesan, breadcrumbs and top with the lettuce.

Nutrition: Calories 107 Total Fat 6.5g Saturated Fat 2.1g Cholesterol 16mg Sodium 360mg Total Carbohydrate 5.4g Dietary Fiber 1.5g Total Sugars 3.3g Protein 6.5g Potassium 372mg

LUNCH

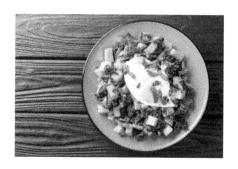

7. Avocado and Kale Eggs

Preparation Time: 10 minutes

Cooking time: 30 minutes

Servings: 3

Ingredients:

- 1 teaspoon ghee

- 1 red onion, sliced

- 4 oz. chorizo, sliced into thin rounds

- 1 cup chopped kale

- 1 ripe avocado, pitted, peeled, chopped

- 4 eggs

- Salt and black pepper to season

Directions:

1. Preheat oven to 370°F.

2. Melt ghee in a cast iron pan over medium heat and sauté the onion for 2 minutes. Add the chorizo and cook for 2 minutes more, flipping once.

3. Introduce the kale in batches with a splash of water to wilt, season lightly with salt, stir and cook for 3 minutes. Mix in the avocado and turn the heat off.

4. Create four holes in the mixture, crack the eggs into each hole, sprinkle with salt and black pepper, and slide the pan into the preheated oven to bake for 6 minutes until the egg whites are set or firm and yolks still runny.

Season to taste with salt and pepper, and serve right away with low carb toasts.

Nutrition:

Kcal 274,

Fat 23g,

Net Carbs 4g,

Protein 13g

8. Bacon and Cheese Frittata

Preparation Time: 10 minutes

Cooking time: 20 minutes

Servings: 3

Ingredients:

- 10 slices bacon 10 fresh eggs

- 3 tablespoon butter, melted

- ½ cup almond milk

- Salt and black pepper to taste

- 1 ½ cups cheddar cheese, shredded

- ¼ cup chopped green onions

Directions:

1. Preheat the oven to 400°F and grease a baking dish with

   cooking spray. Cook the bacon in a skillet over medium

heat for 6 minutes. Once crispy, remove from the skillet to paper towels and discard grease. Chop into small pieces. Whisk the eggs, butter, milk, salt, and black pepper. Mix in the bacon and pour the mixture into the baking dish.

2. Sprinkle with cheddar cheese and green onions, and bake in the oven for 10 minutes or until the eggs are thoroughly cooked. Remove and cool the frittata for 3 minutes, slice into wedges, and serve warm with a dollop of Greek yogurt.

Nutrition:

Kcal 325,

Fat 28g,

Net Carbs 2g,

Protein 15g

9. Spicy Egg Muffins with Bacon & Cheese

Preparation Time: 10 minutes

Cooking time: 20 minutes

Servings: 3

Ingredients:

- 12 eggs

- ¼ cup coconut milk

- Salt and black pepper to taste

- 1 cup grated cheddar cheese

- 12 slices bacon

- 4 jalapeño peppers, seeded and minced

Directions:

1. Preheat oven to 370°F.

2. Crack the eggs into a bowl and whisk with coconut milk until combined. Season with salt and pepper, and evenly stir in the cheddar cheese.

3. Line each hole of a muffin tin with a slice of bacon and fill each with the egg mixture two-thirds way up. Top with the jalapeno peppers and bake in the oven for 18 to 20 minutes or until puffed and golden. Remove, allow cooling for a few minutes, and serve with arugula salad.

Nutrition:

Kcal 302,

Fat 23.7g,

Net Carbs 3.2g,

Protein 20g

10.   Chicken, Bacon and Avocado Cloud Sandwiches

Preparation Time: 10 minutes

Cooking Time: 25 minutes

Servings: 6

Ingredients:

- For cloud bread 3 large eggs

- 4 oz. cream cheese

- ½ tablespoon. ground psyllium husk powder

- ½ teaspoon baking powder

- A pinch of salt To assemble sandwich

- 6 slices of bacon, cooked and chopped

- 6 slices pepper Jack cheese

- ½ avocado, sliced

- 1 cup cooked chicken breasts, shredded

- 3 tablespoons. mayonnaise

Directions:

1. Preheat your oven to 300 degrees.

2. Prepare a baking sheet by lining it with parchment paper. Separate the egg whites and egg yolks, and place into separate bowls. Whisk the egg whites until very stiff. Set aside. Combined egg yolks and cream cheese.

3. Add the psyllium husk powder and baking powder to the egg yolk mixture. Gently fold in.

4. Add the egg whites into the egg mixture and gently fold in.

5. Dollop the mixture onto the prepared baking sheet to create 12 cloud bread. Use a spatula to gently spread the circles around to form ½-inch thick pieces.

6. Bake for 25 minutes or until the tops are golden brown.

7. Allow the cloud bread to cool completely before serving. Can be refrigerated for up to 3 days of frozen for up to 3 months. If food prepping, place a layer of parchment paper between each bread slice to avoid having them getting stuck together. Simply toast in the oven for 5 minutes when it is time to serve.

8. To assemble sandwiches, place mayonnaise on one side of one cloud bread. Layer with the remaining sandwich ingredients and top with another slice of cloud bread.

Nutrition:

Calories: 333 kcal

Carbs: 5g

Fat: 26g

Protein: 19.9g

11. Lemon Chicken Sandwich

Preparation Time: 15 minutes

Cooking Time: 1 hour 30 minutes

Servings: 12

Ingredients:

- 1 kg whole chicken

- 5 tablespoons. butter

- 1 lemon, cut into wedges

- 1 tablespoon. garlic powder

- Salt and pepper to taste

- 2 tablespoons. mayonnaise

- Keto-friendly bread

Directions:

1. Preheat the oven to 350 degrees F.

2. Grease a deep baking dish with butter.

3. Ensure that the chicken is patted dry and that the gizzards have been removed.

4. Combine the butter, garlic powder, salt and pepper.

5. Rub the entire chicken with it, including in the cavity.

6. Place the lemon and onion inside the chicken and place the chicken in the prepared baking dish.

7. Bake for about 1½ hours, depending on the size of the chicken.

8. Baste the chicken often with the drippings. If the drippings begin to dry, add water. The chicken is done when a thermometer, insert it into the thickest part of the thigh reads 165 degrees F or when the clear juices run when the thickest part of the thigh is pierced.

9. Allow the chicken to cool before slicing.

10. To assemble sandwich, shred some of the breast meat and mix with the mayonnaise. Place the mixture between the two bread slices.

11. To save the chicken, refrigerated for up to 5 days or freeze for up to 1 month.

Nutrition:

Calories: 214 kcal

Carbs: 1.6 g

Fat: 11.8 g

Protein: 24.4 g.

12.   Keto Dijon Chicken

Preparation Time: 10 Minutes

Cooking Time: 6 Hours **Servings:** 4

Ingredients:

- 2 lbs. chicken thighs, skinless and boneless

- 3/4 cup of chicken stock

- 1/4 cup of lemon juice

- 2 tablespoon of extra virgin olive oil

- 3 tablespoon of Dijon mustard

- 2 tablespoons of Italian seasoning

- Salt and black pepper- to taste

Directions:

1. Start by throwing all the fixings into the Crockpot and mix them well.

2. Cover it and cook for 6 hours on Low Settings.

3. Garnish as desired.

4. Serve warm.

Nutrition:

Calories 398

Total Fat 13.8 g

Saturated Fat 5.1 g

Cholesterol 200 mg

Total Carbs 3.6 g

Fiber 1 g Sugar 1.3 g

Sodium 272 mg

Potassium 531 mg

Protein 51.8 g

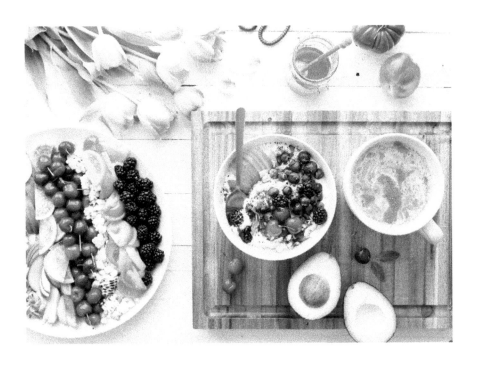

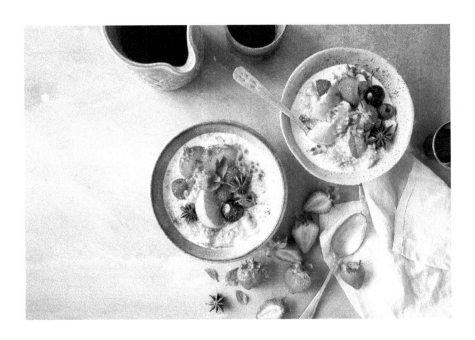

Dinner

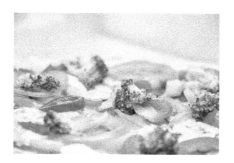

13.   Dill Bell Pepper Bowls

Preparation Time: 10 minutes

Cooking Time: 0 minutes

Servings: 4

Ingredients:

- 2 tablespoons dill, chopped

- 1 yellow onion, chopped

- 1 pound multi colored bell peppers, cut into halves, seeded and cut into thin strips

- 3 tablespoons olive oil

- 2 and ½ tablespoons white vinegar

- Black pepper to the taste

Directions:

- In a salad bowl, mix bell peppers with onion, dill, pepper, oil and vinegar, toss to coat, divide into small bowls and serve as a snack.

Nutrition:

Calories 120

Fat 3 Fiber 4

Carbs 2

Protein 3

14.　　Beef-Stuffed Mushrooms

Preparation Time: 20 minutes

Cooking Time: 25 minutes **Servings: 4**

Ingredients:

- 4 mushrooms, stemmed

- 3 tablespoons olive oil, divided

- 1 yellow onion, sliced thinly

- 1 red bell pepper, sliced into strips

- 1 green bell pepper, sliced into strips

- Salt and pepper to taste 8 oz. beef, sliced thinly

- 3 oz. provolone cheese, sliced

- Chopped parsley

Directions:

1. Preheat your oven to 350 degrees F.

2. Arrange the mushrooms on a baking pan.

3. Brush with oil. Add the remaining oil to a pan over medium heat. Cook onion and bell peppers for 5 minutes. Season with salt and pepper.

4. Place onion mixture on a plate.

5. Cook the beef in the pan for 5 minutes.

6. Sprinkle with salt and pepper.

7. Add the onion mixture back to the pan.

8. Mix well. Fill the mushrooms with the beef mixture and cheese. Bake in the oven for 15 minutes.

Nutrition:

Calories 333 Total Fat 20.3 g Saturated Fat 6.7 g

Cholesterol 61 mg Sodium 378 mg Total Carbohydrate 8.2 g

Dietary Fiber 3.7 g Protein 25.2 g Total Sugars 7 g

Potassium 789 mg

15.   Keto Rib Roast

Preparation Time: 15 minutes

Cooking Time: 3 hours

Servings: 8

Ingredients:

- 1 rib roast

- Salt to taste

- 12 cloves garlic, chopped

- 2 teaspoons lemon zest

- 6 tablespoons fresh rosemary, chopped

- 5 sprigs thyme

Directions:

1. Preheat your oven to 325 degrees F.

2. Season all sides of rib roast with salt.

3. Place the rib roast in a baking pan.

4. Sprinkle with garlic, lemon zest and rosemary.

5. Add herb sprigs on top.

6. Roast for 3 hours.

Let rest for a few minutes and then slice and serve.

Nutrition:

Calories 329 Total Fat 27 g

Saturated Fat 9 g Cholesterol 59 mg

Sodium 498 mg

Total Carbohydrate 5.3 g

Dietary Fiber 1.8 g

Protein 18 g

Total Sugars 2 g

Potassium 493 mg

16.　　**Beef Stir Fry**

Preparation Time: 15 minutes

Cooking Time: 10 minutes

Servings: 4

Ingredients:

- 1 tablespoon soy sauce

- 1 tablespoon ginger, minced

- 1 teaspoon cornstarch

- 1 teaspoon dry sherry

- 12 oz. beef, sliced into strips

- 1 teaspoon toasted sesame oil

- 2 tablespoons oyster sauce

- 1 lb. baby bok choy, sliced

- 3 tablespoons chicken broth

Directions:

1. Mix soy sauce, ginger, cornstarch and dry sherry in a bowl.

2. Toss the beef in the mixture.

3. Pour oil into a pan over medium heat.

4. Cook the beef for 5 minutes, stirring.

5. Add oyster sauce, bok choy and chicken broth to the pan.

6. Cook for 1 minute.

Nutrition:

Calories 247 Total Fat 15.8 g

Saturated Fat 4 g Cholesterol 69 mg

Sodium 569 mg Total Carbohydrate 6.3 g

Dietary Fiber 1.1 g

Protein 25 g

17.   Sweet & Sour Pork

Preparation Time: 15 minutes

Cooking Time: 15 minutes

Servings: 4

Ingredients:

- 1 lb. pork chops

- Salt and pepper to taste

- ½ cup sesame seeds

- 2 tablespoons peanut oil

- 2 tablespoons soy sauce

- 3 tablespoons apricot jam

- Chopped scallions

Directions:

1. Season pork chops with salt and pepper.

2. Press sesame seeds on both sides of pork.

3. Pour oil into a pan over medium heat.

4. Cook pork for 3 to 5 minutes per side.

5. Transfer to a plate.

6. In a bowl, mix soy sauce and apricot jam.

7. Simmer for 3 minutes.

8. Pour sauce over the pork and garnish with scallions before serving.

Nutrition:

Calories 414 Total Fat 27.5 g

Saturated Fat 5.6 g Cholesterol 68 mg

Sodium 607 mg Total Carbohydrate 12.9 g

Dietary Fiber 1.8 g Protein 29 g

Total Sugars 9 g Potassium 332 mg

18.   Tuna Salpicao

Preparation Time: 5 Minutes

Cooking Time: 4 Hours and 10 Minutes

Servings: 3

Ingredients:

- 8 ounce cooked wild-caught tuna, cut into inch cubes

- 4 jalapeno peppers, chopped

- 5 red chilies, chopped

- 1 bulb of garlic, peeled and minced

- 1 teaspoon salt 1 teaspoon ground black pepper

- 1 cup avocado oil

Directions:

1. Place all the ingredients except for tuna in a 4-quart slow

   cooker and stir until mixed.

2. Plug in the slow cooker, shut with lid and cook for 4 hours at low heat setting.

3. Then add tuna and continue cooking for 10 minutes at high heat setting.

4. Serve straightaway.

Nutrition:

Net Carbs: 0.8g;

Calories: 737.6;

Total Fat: 72.1g;

Saturated Fat: 8.6g;

Protein: 20.2g;

Carbs: 1.8g;

Fiber: 0.6g;

Sugar: 1g

Vegetables

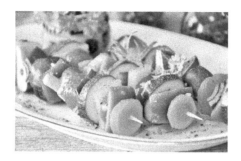

19.   Cauliflower and Egg Rice

Preparation Time: 5 minutes;

Cooking Time: 12 minutes **Servings**: 2

Ingredients

- 8-ounce cauliflower florets, riced

- 2 green onion, sliced

- 1 large egg, beaten

- 1 tbsp. soy sauce

- ½ tsp toasted sesame oil

- Seasoning:

- 1 tbsp. coconut oil

- ½ tsp garlic powder

Directions:

1. Take a large skillet pan, place it over medium-high heat, add coconut oil and riced cauliflower, and cook for 5 minutes until softened.

2. Then add green onions, stir well and cook for 3 minutes until onions are tender.

3. Season with salt, sprinkle garlic over cauliflower, cook for 1 minute until fragrant, then pour in the egg, stir well and cook for 2 minutes until the egg has scrambled to desire level, stirring continuously.

4. Drizzle with soy sauce and sesame oil and Serve.

   Nutrition: 57 Calories; 4 g Fats; 3 g Protein; 1.7 g Net Carb; 0.5 g Fiber

20.   Spinach Zucchini Boats

Preparation Time: 5 minutes

Cooking Time: 10 minutes;

Servings: 2

Ingredients

- 1 large zucchini ¾ cup spinach

- 1 ½ tbsp. whipped topping

- 3 tbsp. grated parmesan cheese

- ½ tsp garlic powder

- Seasoning: ½ tsp salt

- ½ tsp ground black pepper

Directions:

1. Turn on the oven, then set it to 350 degrees F, and let

   preheat.

2. Take a skillet pan, place it over medium heat, add spinach and cook for 5 to 7 minutes or until spinach leaves have wilted and their moisture has evaporated completely.

3. Sprinkle garlic powder, ¼ tsp each of salt and black pepper over spinach, add whipped topping and 2 tbsp. cheese and stir well until the cheese has melted, remove the pan from heat.

4. Cut off the top and bottom of zucchini, then cut it in half lengthwise and make a well by scooping out pulp along the center, leaving ½-inch shell.

5. Season zucchini with remaining salt and black pepper, place them on a baking sheet and roast for 5 minutes.

6. Then fill zucchini evenly with spinach mixture, top with remaining cheese and broil for 3 minutes until cheese has melted.

7. Serve.

Nutrition: 86.5 Calories; 6 g Fats; 4 g Protein; 3.5 g Net Carb;

0.5 g Fiber

21.   Green Beans with Herbs

Preparation Time: 5 minutes

Cooking Time: 7 minutes;

Servings: 2

Ingredients

- 3 oz. green beans 2 slices of bacon, diced

- 3 tbsp. chopped parsley

- 3 tbsp. chopped cilantro 1 tbsp. avocado oil

- Seasoning: ½ tsp garlic powder

- ¼ tsp salt

Directions:

1. Place green beans in a medium heatproof bowl, cover with a plastic wrap, and then microwave for 3 to 4 minutes at high heat setting until tender.

2. Meanwhile, take a medium skillet pan, place it over medium heat and when hot, add bacon and cook for 3 to 4 minutes until crisp.

3. Season bacon with salt, sprinkle with garlic powder and cook for 30 seconds until fragrant, remove the pan from heat.

4. When green beans have steamed, drain them well, rinse under cold water, and then transfer to a bowl.

5. Add bacon and remaining ingredients and toss until well mixed.

6. Serve.

Nutrition: 380 Calories; 33.7 g Fats; 15.2 g Protein; 2.4 g Net Carb; 1.4 g Fiber

22.   lmond Flour Crackers

Preparation time: 15 minutes

Cooking Time: 15 minutes

Servings: 4

Ingredients:

- 1 tablespoon flax meal or whole Psyllium husks

- 2 tablespoons sunflower seeds

- 1 cup almond flour

- 2 tablespoons water

- 1 tablespoon coconut oil

- ¾ teaspoon sea salt or to taste

Directions:

1. Preheat your oven to 350°F.

2. Blend the almond flour with Psyllium, sunflower seeds and sea salt in a food processor or large bowl.

3. If you are blending the ingredients by hand then stir the liquid ingredients into dry ingredients to form a dough ball or if you are using a food processor then pulse in coconut oil and water until dough forms.

4. Place the formed ball of dough on a parchment paper; pressing it flat. Cover with one more parchment paper; rolling the dough out to approximately 1/8 to 1/16" thickness.

5. Put it on a large cutting board; remove the parchment paper on top and cut into 1" squares using a pizza cutter or sharp knife. Sprinkle with the sea salt.

6. Place the cut dough on a large-sized baking sheet; bake in a 350°F oven for 10 to 15 minutes, until edges are crisp and brown. Let cool on a rack and then separate into desired squares.

Nutrition:

149 Calories

13g Total Fat

2.8g Saturated Fat

4.7g Total Carbohydrates

2.9g Dietary Fiber

0.9g Sugars

4.7g Protein

23.   Gluten-Free Bagels

Preparation time: 10 minutes

Cooking Time: 40 minutes

Servings: 6

Ingredients:

- 1 teaspoon baking powder

- ¼ cup Psyllium husks

- ½ cup tahini

- 1 cup water

- ½ cup ground flaxseed

- Sesame seeds for garnish, optional

Directions:

1. Preheat your oven to 375°F in advance.

2. Add the Psyllium husk together with baking powder and ground flaxseeds to a large-sized mixing bowl; whisk until combined well.

3. Add water to the tahini; continue to whisk until combined well.

4. Stir the dry ingredients into the wet; knead until dough ball forms.

5. Form approximately 4" diameter and ¼" thick patties from the prepared batter using your hands. Arrange them on the prepared baking tray and cut a small circle from the center of each round.

6. Sprinkle sesame seeds on the patties.

7. Bake in the preheated oven until turn golden brown, for 35 to 40 minutes.

8. Cut in half and toast just like you do for a normal bagel and then top with your favorite toppings.

Nutrition:

215 Calories

16g Total Fat

2.2g Saturated Fat

14g Total Carbohydrates

12.1g Dietary Fiber

0.2g Sugars

6g Protein

24.   Cabbage with Lemon

Preparation time: 10 minutes

Cooking Time: 30 minutes

Servings: 4

Ingredients:

- 2-3 tablespoons lemon juice, freshly squeezed

- 1/2 head of green cabbage, cut into 8 evenly size wedges, cutting it through the core and stem end

- Fresh ground black pepper and sea salt to taste

- 2 tablespoons olive oil

- Lemon slices, for serving

Directions:

1. Lightly coat a roasting pan with the olive oil or non-stick spray and then preheat your oven to 450°F.

2. Arrange the cabbage wedges on the prepared roasting pan, preferably in a single layer.

3. Whisk the olive oil with lemon juice then brush the top sides of each wedge with the prepared mixture using a pastry brush and generously season with fresh ground black pepper and salt.

4. Carefully turn the cabbage wedges and brush the other side with the lemon juice-olive oil mixture as well then season with pepper and salt.

5. Roast the cabbage until the sides of your wedges is nicely browned, for 12 to 15 minutes.

6. Remove the pan from oven; carefully turning the wedges. Put in the oven again and roast until the cabbage is cooked through and nicely browned, for 10 to 15 more minutes.

7.   Serve hot with more of lemon slices, if desired.

Nutrition:

129 Calories

7.6g Total Fat

1.1g Saturated Fat

8.5g Total Carbohydrates

3g Dietary Fiber

4.5g Sugars

2g Protein

Meat

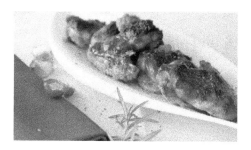

25.   Roast Beef and Vegetable Plate

Preparation Time: 10 minutes

Cooking Time: 10 minutes;

Servings: 2

Ingredients

- 2 scallions, chopped in large pieces

- 1 ½ tbsp. coconut oil

- 4 thin slices of roast beef

- 4 oz. cauliflower and broccoli mix

- 1 tbsp. butter, unsalted

- Seasoning:

- 1/2 tsp salt

- 1/3 tsp ground black pepper

- 1 tsp dried parsley

Directions:

1. Turn on the oven, then set it to 400 degrees F, and let it preheat.

2. Take a baking sheet, grease it with oil, place slices of roast beef on one side, and top with butter.

3. Take a separate bowl, add cauliflower and broccoli mix, add scallions, drizzle with oil, season with remaining salt and black pepper, toss until coated and then spread vegetables on the empty side of the baking sheet.

4. Bake for 5 to 7 minutes until beef is nicely browned and vegetables are tender-crisp, tossing halfway.

5. Distribute beef and vegetables between two plates and then serve.

Nutrition: 313 Calories; 26 g Fats; 15.6 g Protein; 2.8 g Net Carb; 1.9 g Fiber;

26.   **Steak and Cheese Plate**

Preparation Time: 5 minutes;

Cooking Time: 10 minutes;

Servings: 2

Ingredients

- 1 green onion, chopped

- 2 oz. chopped lettuce

- 2 beef steaks

- 2 oz. of cheddar cheese, sliced

- ½ cup mayonnaise

- Seasoning:

- ¼ tsp salt

- 1/8 tsp ground black pepper

- 3 tbsp. avocado oil

Directions:

1. Prepare the steak, and for this, season it with salt and black pepper.

2. Take a medium skillet pan, place it over medium heat, add oil and when hot, add seasoned steaks, and cook for 7 to 10 minutes until cooked to the desired level.

3. When done, distribute steaks between two plates, add scallion, lettuce, and cheese slices.

4. Drizzle with remaining oil and then serve with mayonnaise.

Nutrition: 714 Calories; 65.3 g Fats; 25.3 g Protein; 4 g Net Carb; 5.3 g Fiber;

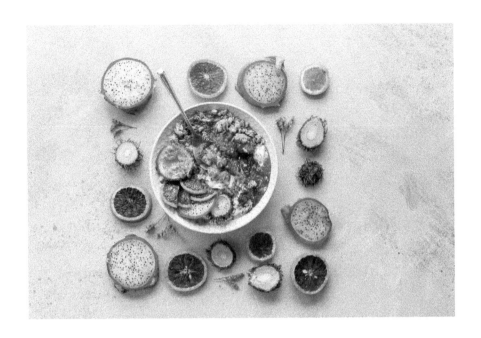

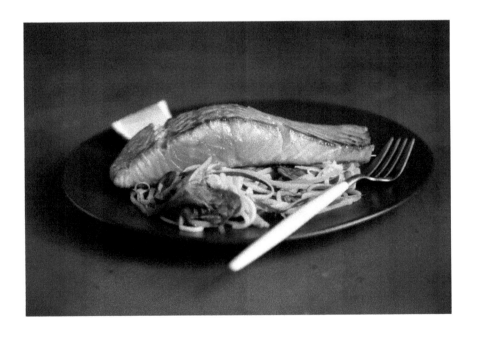

Poultry and Eggs

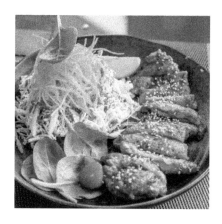

27.   Chicken with Brussel Sprouts

Preparation Time: 120 Minutes

Cooking Time: 40 Minutes

Servings: 8

Ingredients

- 5 pounds whole chicken

- 1 bunch oregano

- 1 bunch thyme

- 1 tbsp. marjoram

- 1 tbsp. parsley

- 1 tbsp. olive oil

- 2 pounds Brussel sprouts

- 1 lemon

- 4 tbsp. butter

Directions

1. Preheat your oven to 450 F.

2. Stuff the chicken with oregano, thyme, and lemon.

3. Make sure the wings are tucked over and behind.

4. Roast for 15 minutes. Reduce the heat to 325 F, and cook for 40 minutes.

5. Spread the butter over the chicken and sprinkle parsley and marjoram.

6. Add the Brussel sprouts. Return to oven and bake for 40 more minutes.

7. Let sit for 10 minutes before carving.

Nutrition Calories 430, Net Carbs 5g, Fat 32g, Protein 30g

28.   Chicken with Grapefruit & Lemon

Preparation Time: 30 Minutes

Cooking Time: 40 Minutes

Servings: 4

Ingredients

- 1 cup omission IPA

- A pinch of garlic powder

- 1 tsp grapefruit zest

- 3 tbsp. lemon juice

- ½ tsp coriander, ground

- 1 tbsp. fish sauce

- 2 tbsp. butter

- ¼ tsp xanthan gum

- 3 tbsp. swerve sweetener

- 20 chicken wing pieces

- Salt and black pepper to taste

Directions

1. Combine lemon juice and zest, fish sauce, coriander, omission IPA, sweetener, and garlic powder in a saucepan.

2. Bring to a boil, cover, lower the heat, and let simmer for 10 minutes.

3. Stir in the butter and xanthan gum. Set aside. Season the wings with some salt and pepper.

4. Preheat the grill and cook for 5 minutes per side.

5. Serve topped with the sauce.

Nutrition Calories 365, Net Carbs 4g, Fat 25g, Protein 21g

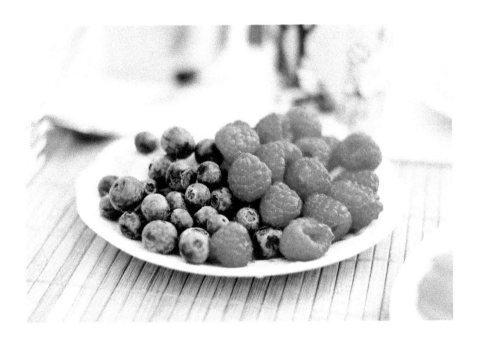

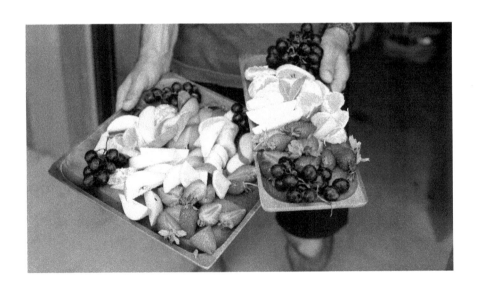

Seafood

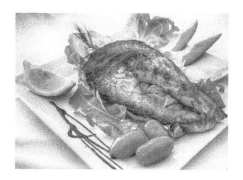

29.　Tuna Salad Pickle Boats

Preparation Time: 10 minutes

Cooking Time: 0 minutes;

Servings: 2

Ingredients

- 4 dill pickles

- 4 oz. of tuna, packed in water, drained

- ¼ of lime, juiced

- 4 tbsp. mayonnaise

- Seasoning:

- ¼ tsp salt

- 1/8 tsp ground black pepper

- ¼ tsp paprika

- 1 tbsp. mustard paste

Directions:

1. Prepare tuna salad and for this, take a medium bowl, place tuna in it, add lime juice, mayonnaise, salt, black pepper, paprika, and mustard and stir until mixed.

2. Cut each pickle into half lengthwise, scoop out seeds, and then fill with tuna salad.

3. Serve.

Nutrition: 308.5 Calories; 23.7 g Fats; 17 g Protein; 3.8 g Net Carb; 3.1 g Fiber

30.   Shrimp Eggs

Preparation Time: 5 minutes

Cooking Time: 0 minutes;

Servings: 2

Ingredients

- 2 eggs, boiled

- 2 oz. shrimps, cooked, chopped

- ½ tsp tabasco sauce ½ tsp mustard paste

- 2 tbsp. mayonnaise

- Seasoning: 1/8 tsp salt

- 1/8 tsp ground black pepper

Directions:

1. Peel the boiled eggs, then slice in half lengthwise and
   transfer egg yolks to a medium bowl by using a spoon.

2. Mash the egg yolk, add remaining ingredients and stir until well combined.

3. Spoon the egg yolk mixture into egg whites, and then serve.

Nutrition: 210 Calories; 16.4 g Fats; 14 g Protein; 1 g Net Carb; 0.1 g Fiber

Snacks

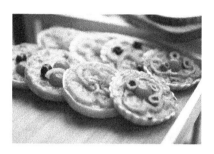

31.Creamy Cheddar and Bacon with Almo

32.   Herbed Cheese Balls

Preparation Time: 30 MIN

Cooking Time: 10 minutes

Servings: 20

Ingredients:

- 1/3 cup grated Parmesan Cheese

- 3 tbsp. Heavy Cream

- 4 tbsp. Butter, melted

- ¼ tsp Pepper

- 2 Eggs

- 1 cup Almond Flour

- ¼ cup Basil Leaves

- ¼ cup Parsley Leaves

- 2 tbsp. chopped Cilantro Leaves

- 1/3 cup crumbled Feta Cheese

Directions:

1. Place the ingredients in your food processor.

2. Pulse until the mixture becomes smooth.

3. Transfer to a bowl and freeze for 20 minutes or so, to set.

4. Shale the mixture into 20 balls.

5. Meanwhile, preheat the oven to 350 degrees F.

6. Arrange the cheese balls on a lined baking sheet.

7. Place in the oven and bake for 10 minutes.

8. Serve and enjoy!

Nutrition:

Calories 60

Total Fats 5g

Net Carbs: 8g

Protein 2g

Fiber: 1g

33. **Cheesy Salami Snack**

Preparation Time: 30 MIN

Cooking Time: 10 minutes

Servings: 6

Ingredients:

- 4 ounces Cream Cheese

- 7 ounces dried Salami

- ¼ cup chopped Parsley

Directions:

1. Preheat the oven to 325 degrees F.

2. Slice the salami thinly (I got 30 slices).

3. Arrange the salami on a lined sheet and bake for 15 minutes.

4. Arrange on a serving platter and top each salami slice with a bit of cream cheese.

5. Serve and enjoy!

Nutrition:

Calories 139

Total Fats 15g

Net Carbs: 1g

Protein 9g

Fiber: 0g

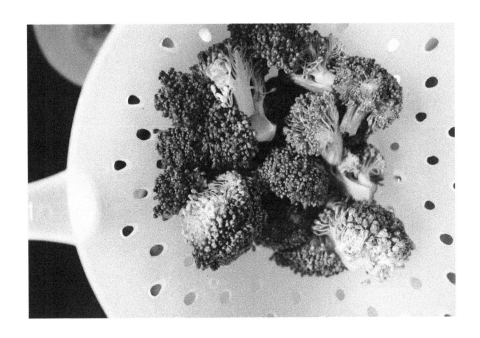

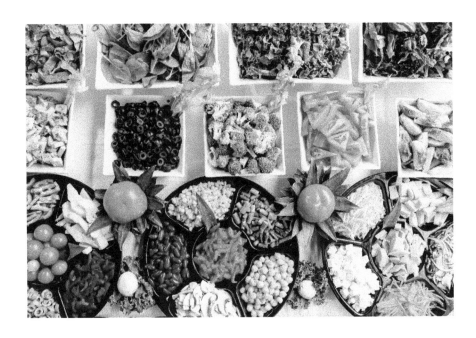

Salads

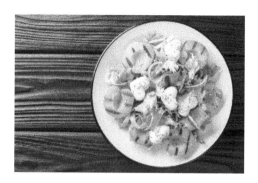

34.   Cauliflower and Cashew Nut Salad

Preparation Time: 10 Minutes

Cooking Time: 5 Minutes **Servings**: 4

Ingredients:

- 1 head cauliflower, cut into florets

- ½ cup black olives, pitted and chopped

- 1 cup roasted bell peppers, chopped

- 1 red onion, sliced

- ½ cup cashew nuts Chopped celery leaves, for

Direction:

1. Add the cauliflower into a pot of boiling salted water. Allow to boil for 4 to 5 minutes until fork-tender but still crisp.

2. Remove from the heat and drain on paper towels, then transfer the cauliflower to a bowl.

3. Add the olives, bell pepper, and red onion. Stir well.

4. Make the dressing: In a separate bowl, mix the olive oil, mustard, vinegar, salt, and pepper. Pour the dressing over the veggies and toss to combine.

5. Serve topped with cashew nuts and celery leaves.

Nutrition: Calories: 298 Cal Fat: 20 g Carbs: 4 g Protein: 8 g Fiber: 3 g

Soups and Stews

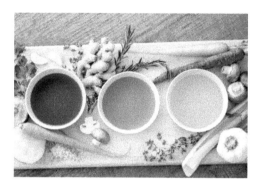

35. Chilled Cucumber Soup

Preparation Time: 15 Minutes

Cooking Time: 0 Minutes **Serving**s: 2

Ingredients:

- 1 cup English cucumber, peeled and chopped

- 1 scallion, chopped

- 2 tablespoons fresh parsley leaves

- 2 tablespoons fresh basil leaves

- ¼ teaspoon fresh lime zest, grated freshly

- 1 cup unsweetened coconut milk

- ¼ cup of water ½ tablespoon fresh lime juice

- Salt and ground black pepper, as required

Direction:

1. Add all the ingredients in a high-speed blender and pulse on high speed until smooth.

2. Transfer the soup into a large serving bowl.

3. Cover the bowl of soup and place in the refrigerator to chill for about 6 hours. Serve chilled.

Nutrition:

Calories: 198 Cal Fat: 10 g

Carbs: 7 g Protein: 9 g

Fiber: 5 g

36.   Mushroom Soup

Preparation Time: 15 Minutes

Cooking Time: 20 Minutes **Servings:** 4

Ingredients:

- 3 tablespoons unsalted butter

- 1 scallion, sliced 1 large garlic clove, crushed

- 5 cups fresh button mushrooms, sliced

- 2 cups homemade vegetable broth

- Salt and ground black pepper, as required

- 1 cup heavy cream

Direction:

1. In a large soup pan, melt the butter over medium heat and sauté the scallion and garlic for about 2–3

minutes. Add the mushrooms cook fry for about 5–6 minutes, stirring frequently.

2. Stir in the broth and bring to a boil.

3. Cook for about 5 minutes.

4. Remove from the heat and with a stick blender, blend the soup until smooth.

5. Return the pan over medium heat.

6. Stir in the cream, salt, and black pepper and cook for about 2–3 minutes, stirring continuously.

7. Remove from the heat and serve hot

Nutrition:

Calories: 195 Cal Fat: 17 g

Carbs: 8 g Protein: 2 g

Fiber: 5 g

DESSERTS

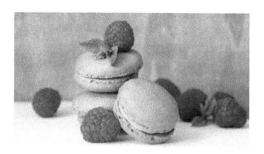

37.   Smoothie with Melon

Ingredients

- 250 g watermelon pulp

- 150 g cherry tomatoes 2 handfuls basil

- Salt pepper from the mill

Preparation steps

1. Roughly dice the melon pulp. Wash and halve the tomatoes. Wash the basil and shake dry. Put everything

together with 100 ml of water in the mixer and puree finely.

2. Depending on the desired consistency, add a little more water. Season to taste with salt and pepper, fill into glasses and serve garnished with basil.

38.   Fruity Herbal Smoothie

Ingredients

- 150 g spinach

- 2 handfuls mixed herbs (e.g. chervil, mint, tarragon, parsley)

- 2 apples

- Orange 1 tsp olive oil

- 500 ml of mineral water

Preparation steps

1. Clean and wash the spinach and herbs and spin dry. Put some herbs aside. Wash, peel, core and cut the apples into large pieces. Squeeze the orange.

2. Puree the spinach, herbs, apple pieces and orange juice in a blender.

3. Add oil and fill up with water. Mix again until foamy and pour the drink into 4 glasses. Serve immediately with straws and the remaining herbs as a garnish.

39.   **Carrot Drink**

Ingredients

- 2 small cloves of garlic

- 800 g bunch of carrots

- flat-leaf parsley

- ½ lemon

- 1 tsp rapeseed oil

Preparation steps

1. Peel the garlic cloves.

2. Wash the carrots thoroughly and cut off the ends.

3. Wash the parsley and shake dry. Squeeze the lemon half.

4. Juice the garlic and 6 carrots in the juicer.

5. Put the parsley and remaining carrots in the juicer and extract the juice.

6. Mix the carrot drink with about 2 tablespoons of lemon juice and the rapeseed oil and enjoy immediately.

40.   **Blackberry and Peach Cocktail**

Ingredients

- 200 g large ripe peaches (1 large ripe peach)

- 200 g blackberry (frozen or fresh)

- 100 ml mineral water (ice cold)

Preparation steps

1. Wash the peach, pat dry, cut in half and remove the stone.

2. Quarter peach;

3. Cut 2-3 thin slices from a quarter and set aside. If necessary, sort fresh berries, rinse and pat dry.

4. Dice the rest of the peach and finely puree with the berries in a blender. (Add frozen fruit, not defrosted.)

5. Put the puree in a glass and fill up with mineral water. Garnish with the peach slices.

Lightning Source UK Ltd.
Milton Keynes UK
UKHW020640260421
382641UK00010B/641